Adrenal Fatigue Solution

Powerful Methods to Boost Your Energy, Improve Metabolism, And Stimulate Your Hormones

Erika Robinson

Table of Contents

Introduction

Adrenal fatigue also known as hypoadrenia is a condition that refers to a group of non-specific symptoms; this is a controversial medical condition as most conventional doctors don't believe this condition exists but naturopaths and complementary doctors believe this condition exists. Even the endocrinology society and other conventional medical associations do not recognize this condition. Till date, this remains a heated topic in the medical community and medically, this condition is referred to as Addison's disease.

This condition was coined "adrenal fatigue" by James Wilson in the year 1998; he was an expert in alternative medicine, a chiropractor and a naturopath. He described this condition as a collection of symptoms that surface when the functions of the suprarenal glands are impaired. He believed that intense and chronic stress is the primary cause of the disease and it appears like chronic infections such as flu, pneumonia or bronchitis.

The suprarenal glands (which are also known as the adrenal glands) are a pair of small glands; they are situated above the kidneys and are part of the endocrine system.

As part of the endocrine system and positioned above the kidneys, the suprarenal glands are a pair of small glands. These glands are also called the adrenal glands.

"Their main function is to produce hormones and one of the hormones produced is cortisol. They help in the production of more than 50 hormones that are responsible for almost every function in the body that are vital for life."

Adrenal glands also play a critical role in the way the body responds to stress; when the brain release a threat signal, the adrenal medulla immediately releases adrenalin hormones and cortisol to help the reaction of the body to the threat, it increases the flow of blood to the brain, heart, and the muscles (the fight-or-flight response). These glands also help in balancing the levels of hormones in the body.

So when a person is under stress for a long period of time; the adrenals are stressed out that they produce little quantity of cortisol, this in turn leads to brain fog, low levels of energy, salt and sugar cravings, depression, dizziness and other symptoms because the adrenal glands and the body cannot cope with the stress level that happens daily.

Apart from production of low levels of cortisol; another complication caused by adrenal fatigue is low production of DHEA, also known as the "parent hormone", and it helps the body to create other important and vital hormones in the body. Naturopaths believe that everybody can experience this condition particular at stressful points in their lives.

CHAPTER ONE: Causes of Adrenal Fatigue

As stated earlier, this is a condition that is characterized by a group of symptoms that are similar to other illnesses; it occurs in people who are under long term physical, emotional and mental stress and most times it is mistaken for an autoimmune disorder.

Those at risk for this condition are shift workers; students who are also working, those who go through much stress at work, people who are under prolonged stress, people with negative thoughts and emotions, single parents, people going through pain and stressful situations like divorce, surgery or mourning over the death of a loved one, busy new parents, insomniacs, sedentary people, people who have poor nutrition and food sensitivities, caregivers, people exposed to toxins and pollutants, and people with the cases of alcohol or drug abuse.

Stress is the biggest cause of adrenal fatigue and it can also lead to chronic fatigue. A study discovered that students who underwent chronic, long-term stress during their final medical exams had impaired function of the hormone cortisol; its awakening response tends to be weak. This stress limited the level of cortisol that rises every morning when people wake up—this help people to feel alert when they wake up; but stress prevents this and makes waking up and alertness difficult even if one had a long hours of sleep.

Another study revealed that students who chronic fatigue syndrome had impairment in the functions of the glands; this affected the female students mostly. Depression can also cause adrenal fatigue; this condition disrupts the levels of cortisol and affects its responses.

CHAPTER TWO: Signs and Symptoms

Signs and symptoms of adrenal fatigue looks like symptoms of other diseases and medical conditions and therefore it is hard to diagnose; this can be due to the fact that the adrenals have a great influence on the whole body because cortisol and other hormones produced affects all parts of the body directly or indirectly.

Dr. Wilson describes how this condition progresses during the day; he says "you wake up and you are can't function without taking a significant amount of caffeine, during the early part of the day you finally feel a burst of energy, then your energy level crashes around 2 p.m. and rises around 6 p.m.; it falls around 9 p.m. again and it is at its highest around 11 p.m. at night".

Some of the signs and symptoms of adrenal fatigue are:

• Brain fog

- Body aches

- Digestive problems

- Poor circulation of blood and numbness in the fingers

- Nervousness

- Respiratory problems, asthma and allergies

- Insulin resistance

- Difficulty getting up in the morning

- Low blood pressure

- Low blood sugar

- Increased fatigue

- Obesity and weight gain (excess fat storage)

- Low levels of energy

- Low libido or decreased sex drive

- Chronic fatigue

- Mood disorders and irritability

- Anxiety

- Depression

- Autoimmune diseases

- Bone loss or muscle loss

- Joint pain

- Hair loss

- Lines in the fingertips

- Skin problems and ailments

- Dry skin

- Imbalanced levels of hormones

- Inability to handle stress

- Frequent urination

- Sleep disorders and disturbances

- Weak response to stress

- Dizziness, faintness and lightheadedness

- Cravings for sweet and salty foods

- A weak or suppressed immune system

CHAPTER THREE:
Diagnosis

Currently, there are no diagnoses for this condition because it mimics the symptoms of other diseases and therefore it is difficult to distinguish it from other medical conditions; and the conventional medical practitioners have refused to recognize it. To them either someone has a normal endocrine system or a total endocrine failure.

Naturopaths believe this condition exists and they see it as a "middle ground" syndrome that has simple cure and easy-to-implement solutions. Dr. Wilson set parameters for this condition but they are non-specific and this has led to the great controversy around this topic.

Despite all these, the fact remains that adrenal fatigue can't be dismissed as false because of the inability of scientists to conduct adequate tests for diagnosis; many people are affected by this condition and they have gotten help with the aid of natural treatment.

Below are tests carried out to diagnose adrenal fatigue; they must be carried out by a scientist who knows and understands the nature of the condition and these tests are rarely definitive.

•   The most commonly carried out test for adrenal fatigue involves checking bodily fluids for high levels of cortisol; saliva is usually used and not blood, this helps the scientist to see abnormal patterns of cortisol which includes an overload or lack of stress response most times. Some scientists also carry out thyroid function test along with this test because the two hormones are interconnected.

• Iris contraction test was developed by Dr. Arroyo in 1924 to diagnose adrenal fatigue and this test can be carried out in the comfort of your home. This test is done by sitting the patient in a dark room; briefly shine a flashlight across the eyes repeatedly and watch the contraction of the eyes.

If the patient has adrenal fatigue; the contraction of the eyes will not last for two minutes and the eyes might even dilate when the flashlight is still on the eyes. This test is based on the theory that when someone has a weakened adrenal function, the iris will not contract properly when exposed to light.

Another test carried out at home to diagnose this condition is the postural low blood pressure test. Blood pressure rises in healthy individuals when they stand up from a laying position; a blood pressure monitor is used to check the blood pressure when laying down and after standing. The result obtained is used to diagnose this condition; if there is no increase in blood pressure or if there is a decrease in blood pressure; it implies that the adrenal glands are weak, damaged or impaired.

- Other tests used to diagnose this condition but are not definitive are Thyroid Stimulating Hormone (TSH) test, neurotransmitter testing, and free T3 (FT3), cortisol/DHEA ratio, total thyroxine (TT4), ACTH challenge, and 17-HP / cortisol ratio.

CHAPTER FOUR:
Treatment

Adrenal fatigue is mainly treated by changes in diet and lifestyle adjustment; there have been huge success rate to the awareness created upon those who don't believe in the existence of this condition and those who don't see food as medicine.

The treatment is also non-invasive and it benefits the whole body in general: it is usually done under the care and supervision of a naturopath.

Treatment involves reducing all kinds of stress on your mind and body; it also involves detoxifying the body to eliminate all toxins and waste products. Negative thinking and emotions are also discouraged; healthy foods and supplements are taken to replenish lost nutrients of the body and to strengthen the immune and endocrine systems.

Treatment procedures mainly involve healthy lifestyle changes, and healthy eating to fight the causes and underlying issues and to also treat the symptoms.

CHAPTER FIVE: Cure

Adrenal fatigue can be cured by following simple rules and they are:

1.   Start an adrenal fatigue diet

2.   Take supplements and herbs

3.   Reduce stress from your life

Start an Adrenal Fatigue Diet

Diet plays a critical role in recovery; there are foods that boost adrenal functions, replenish its energy thereby boosting the overall health of the body.

Before you start this diet, you must first detoxify your body so that the diet will be effective. The body should be detoxified of toxins, chemicals, wastes and unnatural foods that are hard to digest. All these tax the adrenal glands and make them work harder.

Take any of the following daily to detoxify your body; lemon water, ginger and lemon tea, Moringa Tea, crushed garlic, turmeric tea, black seed, aloe Vera gel, or activated charcoal. These are powerful detoxifying agents. Another powerful tool that can detoxify the body and make it new is regular fasting.

After detoxification, it is highly recommended to avoid some foods till you become healthy and recover fully. Some of the foods to avoid are:

• Excess processed carbohydrates are not good and should also be avoided because they can cause inflammation which can worsen the situation. It is known that people crave for high carb foods when stressed; this gives a temporary relief but it makes the adrenal glands work harder. Avoid gluten and too much starch till you recover; this will stop fatigue and increase the levels of your energy.

• Hydrogenated oils; these include soybean oil, canola and corn oil and other vegetable oils; they can cause inflammation even to the adrenal glands. Replace these oils with healthy oils like coconut oil, ghee or organic butter and olive oil.

• Caffeine; it makes it difficult for the adrenal glands to recover and it also affects sleep. Researchers believe that quality sleep and not just quantity can help one overcome this condition. If you must take a caffeinated drink or coffee; make sure it is in the morning before noon and it must be little.

• Microwaved and processed foods; microwaved foods are dangerous; in addition to highly processed foods filled with chemicals, additives, colorings and sweeteners, they wear out and overburden the digestive system by making digestion difficult. They also cause digestive problems and reduce the levels of energy in the body and this leads to fatigue.

• Refined sugars and artificial sweeteners and sweeteners in all its names and forms like aspartame, high fructose corn syrup, and glucose should be avoided, don't take in sugary foods and drinks, they suppress immune response and worsen the situation. You can use natural sweeteners like stevia or honey as alternatives to these products.

• Processed meats; Processed and the chemicals used in processing these meats can stress the adrenal glands and disrupt the levels of hormones in the body. These meats are also loaded with hormones and low in nutrients and all these can throw the body out of balance and cause a lot of health problems. Take organic and grass-fed meat and take proteins in moderation till you recover.

Now, the next step is to replace these unhealthy foods with healthy foods; eat lots of healthy foods to help your body heal quickly. They are dense in vital nutrients; fiber, antioxidants and healthy fats and they have low sugar.

Foods that boost adrenal health and supports their functions are Cordyceps, chaga, olives, coconuts, fermented foods (they are rich in probiotics), healthy fats like avocado, Himalayan sea salt or Celtic, fatty fish caught in the wild (not farmed raise because they are loaded with growth hormones), bone broth, free-range poultry, seaweed and kelp, nuts like almonds and walnuts, seeds like flaxseeds, chia seeds and pumpkin seeds, sprouts, cauliflower, broccoli, Brussels and other cruciferous vegetables.

Proper hydration and regular intake of clean water helps in detoxifying the body; it aids transport of nutrients to the cells of the body, it also helps the body to produce enough digestive juices, this will aid proper digestion and absorption of foods. It also helps in regulating metabolism and body temperature.

You need healthy amounts of proteins; this will help the repair process of the adrenal glands, it will also help to repair the hair, nails, skin and other organs or tissues that have been damaged by this condition. Take plenty organic beans, organic and farm-raised meats, eggs and liver.

Healthy fats like oily fish, nuts and seeds, avocado, coconut and olive oil supplies the body with sufficient energy and serve as precursors for other vital substances made by the body.

Low glycemic index foods are digested slowly and they have little effect on the levels of glucose; it also releases energy that can last for long period of time. Low glycemic index foods include whole grains, soy, lentils and beans; berries and green apples.

CHAPTER SIX:
Supplements and Herbs

Supplements and herbs help the body to heal fast; they help to provide vital nutrients that boost adrenal functions which might be lacking or insufficient in the main meal. They also hasten recovery; fight adrenal fatigue, increase the levels of energy and support a healthy, vibrant and energetic life.

Herbs and supplements to use include:

• Herbs with adaptogenic properties like ashwangandha, holy basil, rosea and Schisandra; they help to balance the levels of cortisol and control the response of the body to stress. These herbs can also alleviate strain on the suprarenal glands.

• Rosemary essential oil helps to decrease high levels of cortisol; it reduces oxidative stress on the cells of the body, you can mix it with lavender oil to make it more effective. You can make an oil-blend and inhale it or add it to your bath water. It can also be used for massage.

- Licorice roots increases the levels of the parent hormone DHEA in the body; it should not be taken for more than 4 weeks at a time; pregnant women and those with heart disease, kidney impairment, and liver problems should not take this herb in particular.

- Lavender oil effectively calms the body and fights stress; it also brings down the levels of cortisol when inhaled.

•   Coenzyme Q10 helps the body to manage stress effectively; it reduces inflammation and fight oxidative stress. Stress causes inflammation in the body and it triggers adrenal fatigue; it increases the coping mechanism of the body to stress, the coping mechanism of the body declines with age or when the production of cortisol is low.

•   Fish oil can reduce the symptoms of adrenal fatigue; it can also reduce the risk of health complications caused by this condition and they include arthritis, skin problems, mental problems, diabetes, immune problems, anxiety, depression, obesity and weight gain, autoimmune diseases and others.

- A deficiency in selenium has been linked with impaired adrenal functions.

- Magnesium prevents and fights adrenal insufficiency and adrenal fatigue.

- Vitamin D boosts adrenal functions and prevents adrenal problems; it also maintains the homeostasis between vital minerals like phosphorous and magnesium and it boosts the density and strength of the bones.

• A deficiency in vitamin B complex has been linked with stress on the adrenal cortex; take quality B-complex supplements especially vitamin B5 and B12.

• Vitamin C can effectively relieve stress, hence it is known as the "stress-busting" nutrients. It also prevents the side effects of stress and reduces the damages done to the body.

Reduce stress

The last step is healing and recovery of adrenal fatigue is to cut down stress; this will restore the functions of your adrenal glands and boosts your overall health. So below are things you can do to ease stress:

• Seek counsel or support when passing through any traumatic experiences like loss of a loved one, divorce, loss of job, financial hardship, heartbreak and other painful experiences of life.

- Make sure you get all the rest you need when tired; get as much rest as possible.

- Relax and meditate often; have time for yourself.

- As an adult; you need not less than 8 hours sleep every night.

- Don't stay up late into the night; have a regular bed time and you should be in bed before 10.

- Avoid negative people, negative emotions, self-talk, and negative energy.

- Laugh and ensure you catch fun everyday

- Eat healthy foods and have a regular food cycle.

- Exercise daily and the exercises should be mild and not strenuous and hard.

Please note that all these should be done under the supervision of a naturopath or physician; pregnant and nursing mothers should be careful with herbs, they shouldn't use any herb or supplement mentioned here unless stated otherwise by a physician or naturopath.

Adaptogens herbs should not be used by pregnant or nursing mothers and only one herb should be used at a time; use one herb before switching to another, do not mix adaptogen herbs. Ashwangandha should be taken in little doses and should not be taken for a long time so that it won't cause problems.

Diabetic patients, those with blood pressure problems, autoimmune diseases, stomach ulcers, thyroid disorders and those that had a recent surgery or have an upcoming surgery should avoid ashwangandha. Holy basil should not be taken for more than six weeks at a stretch; it shouldn't be taken before or after surgery because it can increase one's risk of bleeding.

Pregnant and nursing women should avoid the essential oils mentioned here; lavender oil should not be used with sedatives, and it is safe to consume. Add 3 drops of lavender essential oil to a cup of juice, water or any healthy drink of your choice. Do not ingest rosemary essential oil because it can lead to spasms and vomiting; it can be inhaled or applied topically, mix it with carrier oil like jojoba, coconut, olive or almond oil. The carrier oil should be more than the essential oil or at most it should be a ratio of 50:50.

CHAPTER SEVEN: When to Seek Help

It is time to seek the help of a naturopath when you notice the following:

•   One or more of the symptoms over a long period of time

•   It affects you badly that you find it difficult to go about your daily duties

•   Lifestyle changes, stress reduction and dietary changes have not helped

•   Worse sleeping pattern

- Skin problems like dark patches on the skin or hyperpigmentation

- Dizziness, fainting and general weakness for consecutive days without a cause like a cold or an illness.

- You have stopped menstruating (if you are a lady).

A naturopath will help you with a combination of herbs, supplements and dietary advice; you might also be given hormonal medications or other natural treatments.

An oral dose of hydrocortisone of 20 milligrams can be given to you for routine management of the cortisol while 50 milligrams of the same can be prescribed occasionally. If you don't have access to a qualified naturopath; then you can meet a physician or an endocrinologist.

When all these measures are strictly followed; recovery is guaranteed but it can take months to years. Don't expect fast results because it took years for the adrenal glands to wear out or get weak;

so it will take time for them to recover and build their strength again.

Minor or mild adrenal fatigue requires six to nine months to heal; moderate fatigue need up to 12 to 18 months while severe adrenal fatigue can take up to 2 years to heal.

Printed in Great Britain
by Amazon